Iliana Hernández
Osmany Franco
Dinorah Coffat

Pregnant women living with HIV

Iliana Hernández
Osmany Franco
Dinorah Coffat

Pregnant women living with HIV

Educational intervention for pregnant women living with HIV

ScienciaScripts

Imprint

Any brand names and product names mentioned in this book are subject to trademark, brand or patent protection and are trademarks or registered trademarks of their respective holders. The use of brand names, product names, common names, trade names, product descriptions etc. even without a particular marking in this work is in no way to be construed to mean that such names may be regarded as unrestricted in respect of trademark and brand protection legislation and could thus be used by anyone.

Cover image: www.ingimage.com

This book is a translation from the original published under ISBN 978-620-3-03716-6.

Publisher:
Sciencia Scripts
is a trademark of
International Book Market Service Ltd., member of OmniScriptum Publishing Group
17 Meldrum Street, Beau Bassin 71504, Mauritius
Printed at: see last page
ISBN: 978-620-3-36393-7

Index

Introduction 2

Chapter 1 7
Theoretical and conceptual framework 7

1.1 The formation of human resources in nursing in Cuba 7
1.2 Analysis of nurse technician improvement from the emerging training program.
.... 10

1.3 Advanced education as a paradigm in the improvement of nursing technical personnel 14

1.4 Analysis of care for pregnant women living with HIV/AIDS 19

Objectives 30

Chapter 2 32
Theoretical Methodological Design 32

Theoretical and empirical inquiries: 32

Ethical Considerations: 35

Operationalization of variables 36

Chapter 3 37
Analysis and Research Results. 37

Analysis and research results 46

Conclusions 59

Recommendations 60

Annex 1 61

Annex 2 62

QUESTIONNAIRE 62

INFORMED CONSENT 64

Bibliographical references 65

Bibliography 66

Introduction

Humanity, since its beginnings, has been confronted with plagues that have decimated entire peoples. Throughout history, infectious diseases have played an important role in the well-being of nations. Some have disappeared, in others the causative agents have mutated and new ones have emerged. In ancient times it was leprosy, in the Middle Ages it was the Black Death and today, in the 21st century, it is AIDS.

In the late 1970s, sporadic cases of a rare disease began to be detected, all with a common denominator: *Candida albicans* infection in the mouth and esophagus, accompanied by skin rashes on different parts of the body corresponding to an aggressive form of Kaposi's sarcoma, *Pneumocystis carinnii* pneumonia, and in some cases, neurological damage and unexplained immune system suppression. These cases appeared as far away as Portugal, Haiti, France and the United States, but were not taken into account. [1]

It was on June 5, 1981 that the disease was first officially discussed when *Gottieb, Siegal and Masur*, of the University of California School of Medicine, published in the weekly morbidity and mortality report of the Center for Disease Control in Atlanta, the report of 5 cases of young homosexuals studied at 3 different hospitals in Los Angeles, presenting with *Pneumocystis carinnii* pneumonia. The immune systems of these young men were weakened or almost gone and there was no reason for this.

The fact that homosexual men were the first reported cases of the disease in the United States, despite the fact that cases had already been identified among women, children and the heterosexual population, led to believe that the homosexual lifestyle was directly related to the disease. That is why the first denomination given to the disease was "Gay Cancer", or "Gay Syndrome"; it was also called "Pink Plague",

The "Gay Plague" was later renamed homosexual-related immunodeficiency2.

AIDS found in sexual promiscuity a favorable environment to spread. It coincided with the sexual revolution seen in American society, perhaps influenced by the breakdown of traditional family values, the disenchantment of the Viet-Nam war, the de-dramatization of sexually transmitted diseases thanks to the discovery of penicillin and the massive use of contraceptives.

One of the most discussed theories states that HIV comes from monkeys hunted by humans and that it was transmitted to humans at the beginning of the last century.

It is based on the relatedness of some strains of simian immunodeficiency virus (SIV) and HIV. HIV-1 strains are very similar to chimpanzee SIVcpz, with a sequence homology of about 84%; while HIV-2 is related to Sooti mangabey SIVsm and macaque SIVmac, with homologies of 82-89% and 82-86% respectively. Thus, through the hunting of monkeys as food and the injection of their blood to man in certain tribes, in search of rejuvenation, the disease could be acquired. Once a man was infected in some region of the African forest, its passage to the urban world and its spread could be explained by the demographic and social phenomena that took place on that continent.

HIV infection is currently considered incurable, although there are antiretroviral drugs that are capable of containing the infection. In developed countries, those infected can lead a completely normal life, like a chronically ill person, without developing AIDS thanks to treatment. However, in other parts of the world, where these drugs are not available, those infected develop AIDS and die within a few years of diagnosis.

HIV is the virus that causes Acquired Immunodeficiency Syndrome (AIDS). It is a member of the Retrovirus family and the Lentivirus subfamily, has an outer envelope and a genetic message composed of RNA and also an enzyme (Retroversotranscriptase) that converts the virus RNA into DNA in the host cell.

Today, 25 vaccine trials are being carried out simultaneously to confront HIV/AIDS. One of the most eagerly awaited has been the GP120 vaccine, from the company VaxGen, which attempts to modify the action of the antigen of that name, which is found on the surface of the cell and which, under normal conditions, allows HIV to invade the organism.

Cuba has been working on obtaining an immunogen capable of preventing HIV infection. The work has been focused on 3 fundamental variants of vaccines: synthetic peptides, recombinant proteins and naked DNA vaccines. A first vaccine produced with synthetic peptide technology was tested in humans in 1998, in phase I studies, making Cuba the fourth country in the world to carry out studies of this type. The vaccine consisted of a multi-epitope polypeptide containing V3 regions of go120 from several different virus isolates. Although somewhat reactogenic, the polypeptide was able to induce antibody response and lymphoproliferative response in the group of vaccinated individuals.

Cuba, knowing about the existence of AIDS in the United States and some developed countries, began to worry about it and sent prestigious researchers to learn more about the infection and decided to put into practice a series of measures to prevent the penetration and propagation of this syndrome in the national territory: The entry into the country of blood products from countries where the existence of this syndrome was known is suspended, an epidemiological surveillance system is put into effect in hospitals with the mandatory reporting of cases of recurrent pneumonia and Kaposis Sarcoma, a network of laboratories for diagnosis is created in the country, The HIV/AIDS Prevention Program was put into effect in Cuba, all blood donations and the most at-risk population were screened, and in 1986, the entire prevalence of HIV-infected internationalists returning from African countries and others returning from abroad began to be admitted to hospitals. [4]

The "Los Cocos" Sanatorium in Santiago de las Vegas, Havana City, was created in 1986, as a result of the country's need to investigate the behavior of a little-known epidemic and prevent the spread of HIV in the national territory. It was the only center of its kind responsible for the admission of all persons infected with HIV, most of whom were returning from abroad on Internationalist Missions, for which reason it was initially run by the medical services of the Revolutionary Armed Forces.

At present, HIV/AIDS patients are cared for on an outpatient basis, i.e. care is provided through the municipal care centers for these patients in conjunction with the doctors and nurses of the family medical office, who provide them with follow-up care and help them improve their quality of life.

In our country, as part of the Maternal and Infant Program, the Ministry of Public Health has been concerned about the follow-up of women living with HIV/AIDS, since there are a number of them who, in spite of the disease, have decided to have a child after medical advice and the stability of the results of the complementary tests (determination of lymphocytes). Therefore, at the Eusebio Hernández Maternal Hospital, comprehensive care for pregnant women living with HIV/AIDS has been centralized, with good results. Nevertheless, different

problematic situations have been identified in the management of patients by the nursing staff in primary health care, such as the following:

> ➤ Difficulty in the management of drug therapy.

> ➤ Difficulty in nutritional follow-up of pregnant women

> ➤ Difficulty in preparing the patient for the moment of delivery.
> ➤ Lack of knowledge of the drug therapy to be administered to the neonate.

For all these   reasons, we formulate the following **scientific problem** as follows

The following question is: How to design a course to prepare the nursing staff working in Primary Health Care in the management of pregnant patients living with HIV/AIDS, together with the above-mentioned background, from this scientific problem it is recognized as an **object of research**

research: professional performance and as a   **field of research:**

preparation of nurses in the   management of pregnant patients living with HIV/AIDS.

Chapter 1

Theoretical and conceptual framework

1.1 The formation of human resources in nursing in Cuba

The documentary analysis of the historical background of the formation of nursing human resources goes back to the care provided by nuns, the contributions made by Florence Nigthingale to nursing as a profession.

The formation of human resources in nursing was analyzed by the author and subdivided the formation of human resources for this purpose: conquest, war of independence, North American intervention, suedorrepublic and the different periods after the triumph of the revolution, taking as indicators the formation of human resources according to the study plans. In 1522 the first hospital was built in Santiago de Cuba, which served as a clinic and took care of the needy. During this period, the city council demanded to examine those who practiced medicine without a degree, the habilitation was easily granted to healers and amateurs.

From the year 1762 it is known that Doña María Chávez, Doña Rita Leal and later Doña María Candelaria Blanco worked in the women's ward of the Ermita San Francisco de Paula, and in 1673 the nursing regulations were approved. At the time of the first American intervention, a group of American nurses: Miss Quintard and Miss Sarah S Henry were appointed as special hospital inspectors to establish practical nursing schools in Cuba. In 1899, the Nuestra Señora de las Mercedes Hospital was inaugurated in Havana.

the 1st preparatory school for nursing students. From 1900 onwards, different hospitals were founded

In 1899, the first nursing school was created at the Nuestra Señora de las Mercedes Hospital, where 7 students were admitted, who did not mind the censorship of the society. In the year 1900 by military order the nursing profession was created with official character, at this time nursing reached high levels due to the introduction of modern concepts based on the principles elaborated in the previous century by Florence Nightingale.

The following subjects were taught during the nursing course: nursing care, pharmacology and therapeutics, semiology, pediatrics, dietetics, surgical pathology, medical pathology, neurology and psychiatry, anatomy and physiology, microbiology, health education, gynecology, obstetrics, supervision and administration, different specialties such as: otorhinolaryngology, ophthalmology.

After the revolutionary triumph, the need to develop an educational system that would guarantee the training of human resources arose. The National Directorate was created, curricula were drawn up, degrees such as those of midwives were validated, and complementary courses in nursing and pediatrics were given.

In 1976, 4-year university nursing curricula began to be developed for intermediate technician graduates and 5-year curricula for 12th grade graduates. Between that year and 1980, the following activities were developed that allowed to improve the quality of the training of nursing human resources and that were analyzed by Magaly Castro:

- ➢ Common trunks were established while preserving the exit profiles.
- ➢ Curricula and syllabi improved
- ➢ Production of textbooks and auxiliary media
- ➢ Methodological guides governing the administrative teaching process were developed.
- ➢ The qualification of the teaching staff was improved and upgraded.
- ➢ High school and university education were articulated
- ➢ The political and sports movement was boosted
- ➢ Only three levels of technical education were left: high school, specialization, and university.

In the 80's the curricula and the programs of the nursing auxiliary courses to become technical nurses were improved, in addition, the level of demand to study nursing was raised and a group of requirements had to be met, such as: [5]

- ➢ Have obtained a comprehensive evaluation
- ➢ Meeting the social requirements to be a health care worker
- ➢ Index higher than 85 points
- ➢ Have no physical or mental handicaps
- ➢ Maintain a proper appearance and appearance
- ➢ Maintain willingness to provide services in any part of the country and other countries.
- ➢ Commit to conduct in accordance with socialist medical ethics.

➢ Be considered suitable in the personal interview process, which includes
a previous analysis of the student's cumulative file.

➢ To be considered fit in the medical examinations.

As a result of the transformations of the National Health System, in the 1987-1988 academic year, a new plan of studies for the Bachelor's Degree in Nursing for Regular Day Course was initiated, thus increasing the number of university nurses who entered higher studies from pre-university institutes with a 12th grade level, and with the prior approval of the entrance exams. In 2001, due to the deficit of nurses in the capital of the country, the emerging training plan for nurses was developed, with a study plan that was in force until 2003. From that moment on, a new pedagogical model was designed, with a duration of 5 years and with three intermediate exit profiles: basic nurse: 1 year, higher technician: 2 more years, and graduate: 2 more years.

The following is an analysis of the behavior of nurses' self-improvement.

1.2 Analysis of nurse technician improvement from the emerging training program.

The documentary analysis of the work of Dr. Omayda Urbina Laza about: Professional profiles, functions and competencies of nursing personnel in Cuba, it addresses the care functions that nursing technicians should develop, among them, the author highlights [6]

3. Comply with the principles of asepsis, antisepsis and biosafety standards, according to the performance contexts.

4. Comply with ethical principles.

5. Participate in the preparation, analysis and discussion of the health situation of its population, detecting vulnerable groups, risk factors and implementing actions aimed at their reduction and/or elimination.

6. Execute actions that provide solutions to the health problems identified in the health situation analysis.

7. Execute actions included in the health programs that provide solutions to the problems of their community.

8. Perform the Nursing Care process, as a scientific method of the profession.

8.1. Record in the medical record all available information on the problems identified in individuals, family and community.

9. Plan and implement health promotion and health promotion activities for individuals, families and communities.

11. Execute disease prevention and protection activities for individuals, families and the community.

14. Perform nursing techniques and procedures within the scope of their competence.

15. Apply alternative medicine techniques and procedures within the scope of their competence.

17. Plan and execute actions aimed at environmental control and the achievement of a healthy environment.

18. Promote intersectoral and multidisciplinary collaboration in the management of health care for the population.

19. Detect educational needs and elaborate health education programs in the search for improvement of quality of life.

20. Train health brigadistas and volunteer groups to participate in health

promotion.

21. Perform nursing actions in emergency and disaster situations.

22. Identify, in your community or emergency services, signs and symptoms of complications, for example: hypo- and hyperglycemia, *shock*, convulsions, bleeding, inform the physician and take action as appropriate.

26. Prepare patients for clinical laboratory investigations (blood count, glycemia, blood culture, urine, stool, stool, culture of secretions, exudates, hemogasometry, blood count, creatinine, leukogram) and special clinical investigations (colon by enema, simple urinary tract, urogram, spinal X-ray, rectosigmoidoscopy, colonoscopy, myelography, laparoscopy, arteriography, lumbar puncture, gynecological ultrasound, *Douglas* sac puncture, amniocentesis and others).

27. Comply with medical treatment.

28. Perform the preparation and administration of drugs by different routes.

29. Perform care for the deceased.

30. Identify reactions produced by drugs and other substances, communicate it and comply with indicated actions.

31. Identify signs and symptoms of surgical emergency such as: evisceration, bleeding, hypovolemic *shock*, wound dehiscence, communicate and take action.

33. Identify signs and symptoms of food or drug intoxication, communicate it and comply with indications.

34. Identify signs and symptoms of alterations of hydromineral and acid-base balance, communicate them and comply with indications.

35. Identify signs and symptoms of complications, e.g., hypo- and hyperglycemia, *shock*, seizures, bleeding, communicate and comply.

37. Perform the preparation and administration of drugs by different routes.

38. Identify adverse reactions to drugs and other substances, stop the application, communicate it and comply with indications.

The changes that are taking place at the international level in the field of health, in the Cuban National Public Health System, in the curriculum and programs of the different subjects of the nursing career reveal a permanent process of renewal and updating of knowledge to carry out the process of development of professional skills, the improvement must then be in accordance with the needs of the nurse to provide a solution to the professional problems he/she faces in his/her performance.

The concept of improvement has been defined in the theory of Advanced Education as "Directed to labor resources with the purpose of updating and perfecting the current and/or future professional performance, addressing insufficiencies in training, or completing knowledge and skills not previously acquired and necessary for performance. It is an organized, systemic process, but its execution is not regulated, it generally does not accredit for performance, it only certifies certain contents".

The author assumes as professional improvement, the "set of teaching-learning processes that enable university graduates to acquire and continuously improve the knowledge and skills required for a better performance of their responsibilities and job functions" (Añorga, J.). (Añorga, J. et al., 1995) [7] and as improvement the one offered in her doctoral thesis (María Luisa Santiesteban, 2003) who, thinking about it in terms of elementary school principals, defines improvement as a "system of conscious actions, with a continuous, systemic, person-logical and evaluable character, which, based on individual commitments, motivations and the theoretical-practical experience of principals, enables them to achieve their aspirations and eradicate difficulties in their professional performance, achieving a knowledge of being that satisfies the new demands of the Cuban elementary school of the 21st century8.

The technical nurse improves himself/herself through post-basic courses, teaching categorization as a Technical Teaching Assistant (TTA), his/her own self-improvement and self-preparation, which must be a logical necessity that starts with the

professional problems he/she faces during his/her professional performance.

1.3 Advanced education as a paradigm in the improvement of nursing technical personnel.

Based on the documentary analysis of the improvement of human resources, the author carried out an analysis of the theory of Advanced Education as a paradigm of professional and human improvement.

Its maximum exponent is Dr. Julia Añorga, in the glossary of terms of Advanced Education it is conceptualized as "Alternative Educational Paradigm ¨ that studies and systematizes the process of improvement of human beings to provide them with new knowledge, skills, habits, feelings, attitudes, abilities, values, behavior and health, empowering them for the transformation and production of knowledge in the human beings participating in each educational paradigm, the growing motivation, the creative activity, the collective conscience, the responsibility with the acquired knowledge and abilities generating conscious potentialities of human growth to transform reality, making viable the elevation of professionalism, the cooperative ethical conduct and the personal and social satisfaction7.

The antecedents of Advanced Education are based on figures that constitute paradigms of our country such as José Martí, José de la Luz y Caballero, Félix Varela who contributed to develop the thinking of the young people of the XVII and XIX centuries, their pedagogical thoughts are advanced for the time in the search for solutions for the improvement of society, in the need for instruction and education, the needs for the improvement of men.

The Advanced Education having as object of study the professional and human improvement of the resources and its historical projective movement produces technologies directed to the improvement of the human resources, consolidation of values, feelings, having as objective:

> Individual: spiritual and professional

> Social: efficiency and productive quality

Advanced education encompasses the improvement for all graduates of the different levels of education, in relation to the cognitive sphere of individuals, the affective sphere, which is fundamental to promote developmental learning, allowing individuals from any position to enjoy their professional activity and perform it with the required quality according to the professional problems they face in their professional activity.

When analyzing the technologies of Advanced Education, we find the Systems of Improvement which have been assumed by nursing professionals as forms of improvement, which have a multifaceted, interdisciplinary character.

The forms of Advanced Education are in function of raising the preparation of men to transform their environment and satisfy their needs and those of the society that surrounds them, among them we have:

Common to all human resources. Workshops, Seminars, Courses, Self-improvement, Conferences, Qualifications, Training, etc.

Foruniversitygraduates:Professional improvement (postgraduate training, diploma courses, etc.) and Academic Training (Specialty, Master's, and Doctorate).

All the forms that have been developed and those to be developed are based on the needs and interests of health institutions and nursing human resources to solve the problems of teaching and nursing practice and thus provide higher quality care, and also promotes a high motivation of these resources because they can produce more scientifically and have a better personal satisfaction.

The forms that have been used in nursing for the development of these resources have been in correspondence with the levels that exist in Cuba, which are the following:

--------Technical Level.

-------Post basic level.

-------Professional level (university)

Advanced Education also proposes a system of principles that are evidenced in the improvement of human resources and that will be explained in its implication in the design of the course for the care of pregnant women with HIV/AIDS, such as:

- ✓ Relationship between social belonging, objectives, motivation and communication.

- ✓ Relationship between forms, technologies and their accreditation.

- ✓ Relationship between theory and practice and the formation of values.

- ✓ Linkage between the system approach and its branch,

sectoral, territorial and community expressions.

- ✓ Conditionality between undergraduate, basic and specialized training.
- ✓ Link between creativity and the quality of the result.
- ✓ Linking the scientific character of the research content and cognitive independence and the production of new knowledge.

Curriculum designs provide the necessary tools to sufficiently develop health actions, thus strengthening essential knowledge and skills, i.e., what they **KNOW** and **KNOW HOW TO DO**. This level of analysis indicates that there is a goal in this research aimed at training researchers in the area of comprehensive care for people with HIV/AIDS with the intention of improving the professional competencies of health professionals who interact with these subjects. [4]

In this regard, it is worth mentioning that Cuba has ventured into educational models in the field of Tropical Diseases through various designs of master's degrees and other postgraduate training at the Institute of Tropical Medicine: Dr. Pedro Kouri (IPK), approved by the Higher Institute of Medical Sciences of Havana and the MES. Taking into consideration that the previous designs respond to general topics such as: Epidemiology, Infectology and Tropical Diseases, Microbiology, Virology and Parasitology, and that these do not address comprehensive care for people with HIV/AIDS, only that in their curriculum appears a module designed for learning about Retroviruses and their classification, in Lentivirus that includes HIV, and Oncoviruses that include HTLD1 and HTLD2, which give rise to AIDS-related tumors and neoplasms. [4]

Academic components of the Graduate System.

Professional Development: Includes short courses, training courses and

The aim is to increase the effectiveness and efficiency of the

professional   work and their cultural training.

Postgraduate Academic Training: These are the Specialties of

Postgraduate, Master's and Doctoral Programs. It aims at postgraduate training with high professional competence and advanced capabilities for scientific, technological and humanistic research, which allows the university graduate to reach a qualitatively superior level from the professional and scientific point of view, which is recognized with an official title of Scientific Degree.

Course: Enables basic and specialized training of graduates.

The course includes the organization of a set of contents. Those that address relevant research results or transcendental aspects of updating may be taught as postgraduate courses.

Training: Enable basic and specialized training for the

university graduates, particularly in the acquisition of skills and abilities and in

the assimilation and introduction of new techniques and technologies.

Diploma: Enabling specialized training of graduates

The program provides for the acquisition of knowledge and the development of

skills in aspects of a particular area of science or art.

Master's degree: A postgraduate training process that provides graduates with

university students have a deep mastery of research methods, a broad scientific

culture and advanced knowledge in a field of knowledge, developing skills for

teaching, research and development work.

Doctorate: A postgraduate training process that provides students with the university graduates a deep and broad knowledge in a field of knowledge, as well as scientific maturity, innovativeness, creativity to solve and direct the solution of problems of scientific character in an independent manner and allowing to obtain a scientific degree.

1.4 Analysis of care for pregnant women with HIV/AIDS.

Studies published in the world show that it is possible to reduce mother-to-child transmission of HIV to levels of 2% when preventive interventions are carried out in time at each of the gestational stages, without the application of the same, it can be as high as 25.5%.

In developed countries, the wide implementation of interventions resulted in a significant reduction in the incidence of AIDS cases in children. Studies conducted in the United States, Europe, Africa and Asia confirmed the efficacy of zidovudine in mother-to-child transmission, even when the gestational intervention was performed late or when it was only administered to the newborn.

Other studies have shown that elective cesarean section is a protective factor for mother-to-child transmission regardless of the application of zidovudine treatment. It is vitally important to take viral load into account since its increase has been recognized as one of the main factors associated with mother-to-child transmission and a determining factor in intrapartum transmission.

Recent studies demonstrate the importance of discerning between the use of antiretroviral drugs as prophylaxis for the prevention of mother-to-child transmission or the use of antiretroviral drugs as treatment in pregnant women who require it due to their clinical and immunological condition.

On the other hand, it is considered of great importance to take into account that the risk of acquiring infection increases between 12-26% in children who are breastfed, the longer they are breastfed the higher the risk, being considerable after three months of age, where the mother's viral load figures play an important role.

The number of HIV-infected women is increasing worldwide. In Cuba, the HIV infection rate varied from 7.29 per 1,000,000 inhabitants in 1987 to 7.29 per 1,000,000 inhabitants in 2000.

As of February 1996, asymptomatic seropositives numbered 735 (60%), AIDS cases 153 (13%) and deaths 324 (27%) by age group, seropositives aged 15 to 24 years had a rate of 17.3 per 1000 000 inhabitants aged 15 to 24 years.

Health services should offer HIV screening tests and advice on safe sex practices, especially aimed at adolescents and young adults, since they are the group where the number of infected people is increasing most rapidly.

The major responsibility of the obstetrician/gynecologist is to reduce the risk of vertical sexual transmission.

Currently, the possibility of reducing the risk by means of a therapeutic regimen based on three elements has been demonstrated.

1- Zidovudine (ZDV) from 14 weeks gestation until the end of gestation.

2-Intravenous Zidovudine (ZDV) during labor and delivery

3-Oral Zidovudine (ZDV) to the newborn during the first 6 weeks of life.

The American College of Obstetrics and Gynecology takes viral load into account and has chosen 1000 copies/ml as the threshold above which it recommends cesarean section for prevention of vertical transmission. If a decision is made to perform a scheduled cesarean section, it is advised that it be performed at 38 weeks gestation.

Treatment with intravenous Zidovudine should be started 3 hours before surgery. Peri-operative antimicrobial prophylaxis can be administered. If the viral load is less than 1000 copies/ml at 36 weeks of gestation, the risk of peri-natal transmission is equal to 2% lower, even if the delivery is transvaginal, if the woman chooses to have a cesarean section, her decision should be respected. If it is not possible to determine the viral load, delivery should be by cesarean section.

Breast-feeding is not advisable because cases of infection through breast milk have been demonstrated.

So far, no significant influence of pregnancy on HIV disease progression has been documented.

The passive transfer of maternal antibodies to the fetus and their persistence in the newborn's blood for 18 months means that, in the absence of symptoms and specific positive tests, it may be impossible to determine whether the child has been infested until 18 months of age.

In Cuba, since 1986, when the serological screening for HIV infection began in the country, the study and follow-up of children born to HIV-positive mothers has been implemented from the clinical and laboratory point of view.

In 1990 they began the direct clinical trial for the early diagnosis of HIV infection in children carrying out the internationally recommended schemes for the interpretation of the results and the time needed in order to be certain whether or not there was transmission of HIV infection from the mother to the child.

In 1987, a strategy for the prevention of mother-to-child transmission of HIV was implemented, which consisted of carrying out HIV tests to determine the serological status of pregnant women during their first prenatal visit.

In Cuba, there are few pediatric cases of HIV/AIDS infection due to the prevention and control program of perinatal transmission implemented in the country since 1989.

To date, there are 203 live births to 195 HIV-positive mothers, taking into account that there are 8 mothers who have given birth twice.

- Infested children24/203 (11.8%)
- Non-infested children 144/203 (70.9%)
- In studies35/203 (17.2%)

Of the 24 infested cases, 10 were treated with tritherapy, 6 were asymptomatic and 8 died.

Since 1993, the number of children born to HIV-positive mothers has increased as a result of the spread of HIV/AIDS among women of reproductive age and the number of these women who choose to have children despite being HIV-positive.

The health policy, as long as the couple accepts it and gives their authorization, suggests the termination of the pregnancy.

The program establishes that all HIV-positive pregnant women detected in their health area will be tested for HIV in order to know their serological status at their first prenatal visit. These pregnant women who wish to have their child after 14 weeks of pregnancy will receive treatment with zidovudine (AZT) 500mg until they are ready to have their baby.

The delivery will be by cesarean section as contemplated in the program in order to avoid routes of contagion such as contact with the mother's vaginal secretions, as well as the suspension of breastfeeding, which is another route of contagion by offering artificial breastfeeding.

The newborn is followed up 8 hours after birth, receiving zidovudine (AZT) syrup at a dose of 2 mg per kg of body weight every 6 hours during the first 6 weeks of life.

Considering that the work of the family physician and nurse rests on the pillars of health promotion and prevention, it is of vital importance to manage the HIV-positive pregnant woman, taking into account the preparation of the nursing staff as a member of the basic health group.

Once the pregnant woman has been identified, the couple is alerted, taking into account whether or not the patient has received treatment with AZT, offering facilities to proceed with the termination of pregnancy as long as it is accepted by the couple voluntarily. If the couple's response is affirmative, the pregnancy will be terminated; otherwise, prenatal follow-up will be given, incorporating AZT at 14 weeks of pregnancy and the child in the first 6 weeks of life and follow-up by specialized consultation at the Pedro Kouri Institute.

Health services should offer HIV screening tests and advice on safe sex practices, especially aimed at adolescents and young adults, since they constitute the group where the number of infected people is increasing most rapidly.

The major responsibility of the obstetrician/gynecologist is to reduce the risk of vertical sexual transmission.

<u>General principles</u>

Studies published in the world show that it is possible to reduce maternal infant transmission of HIV to levels of 2% when preventive interventions are carried out in time at each of the gestational stages. In the absence of preventive measures, the risk of a newborn contracting the virus from an infected mother ranges from 15-25% in developed countries to 25-35% in developing countries. This difference is mainly due to feeding practices; breastfeeding is more frequent and is usually maintained longer in underdeveloped countries than in the industrialized world.

According to the results obtained by the protocol, the reduction of mother-to-child transmission (MTCT) is possible, even when the viral load (VL) was below 1000 copies/ml. Studies carried out in the United States, Europe, Africa and Asia confirmed the efficacy of Zidovudine (AZT) in reducing mother-to-child transmission, even when the intervention was performed late in pregnancy or when it was administered only to the newborn.

Other studies have shown that elective cesarean section is a protective factor against mother-to-child transmission of HIV and reduces the risk of mother-to-child transmission, independent of the effects of Zidovudine treatment.

In Cuba, since 1986, when the serological screening of HIV infection began in Cuba, the study of children born of HIV-positive mothers has been implemented, both from the clinical and laboratory point of view. For this purpose, indirect antibody detection assays were used during the first years. Since 1990, the polymerase chain reaction has been used as the recommended direct test for the early diagnosis of HIV infection in children, following the internationally recommended schemes for the interpretation of the results and the time needed to determine with certainty whether or not there was transmission of HIV infection from mother to child.

In 1987, a strategy for the prevention of mother-to-child transmission of HIV was implemented, which consisted of HIV testing to determine the serological status of pregnant women at their first prenatal visit.

In 1994, antiretroviral treatment with Zidovudine was introduced in the first trimester and elective cesarean section, when the pregnancy is at term.

The newborn is prescribed treatment with Zidovudine from the first 6 hours after birth. For 6 weeks, breastfeeding is prohibited and artificial lactation is indicated, which is ensured through the mechanisms established for this purpose.

<u>Factors contributing to the reduction of mother-to-child transmission.</u>

1- Promotion of interventions that reduce maternal viral load.

2- Use of ART to try to keep viral load below 1000 copies/ml until the end of gestation.

3- Rapid delivery, in case it is unavoidable. 4- Adequate assistance to the mother/child binomial.

5- Prohibition of breastfeeding.

If a diagnosis of HIV infection is made during pregnancy, the patient should be evaluated by a multidisciplinary assistance team specialized in the management of AIDS, which guarantees clinical follow-up and prenatal care.

The main objectives of the management of the HIV-positive pregnant woman include the following

1- Prevent mother-to-child transmission.

2- Delay progression to the asymptomatic stage.

3- Avoid opportunistic infections

4- Treat the complications of immunodeficiency. 5-

To assess the history of ARV treatment.

6- Treatment of STIs.

7- Conduct referral counseling for breastfeeding suppression.

8- Provide reproductive health counseling (effects of pregnancy on their clinical immune status, need for ARV use to prevent MTCT, importance of adherence to ARV therapy, prevention of other sexually transmitted infections (STIs), importance of

maintaining safe sexual practices and prevention of drug dependence during pregnancy).

9- Conduct a complete medical history, including questioning about risk practices.

10- Peri-natal medical history: previous pregnancies and deliveries, occurrence of complications.

11- Complete physical examination, paying special attention to those symptoms and signs that may be associated with HIV (advise the patient to seek immediate care if new symptoms such as diarrhea, shortness of breath, persistent fever, etc. appear).

12- Apply the recommended vaccination schedule according to the established schedule.

13- Supplement pregnancy with iron and folic acid.

14- Prioritize dental care in their health area.

15- Ensure adequate nutritional status, with hypocaloric and hyperproteic diet (4000-4500 cal).

16- A minimum of 8 check-ups will be performed for each pregnant woman and as many as required on an individual basis.

17- Surgical sterilization will be performed only if authorized. 18- Breastfeeding will not be provided.

HIV-positive pregnant women will be attended at the three levels of health care, where they will be followed up according to the level of care, with viral load and CD4 tests, evaluation by the specialized AIDS team, recommended studies and prophylaxis of opportunistic infections.

The use of ARVs in HIV-positive pregnant women is divided into two stages, during pregnancy and during cesarean section and/or delivery (to be summarized). In the second stage of treatment, Zidovudine (PACTG-076) will be administered intravenously three hours before the start of elective cesarean section until the umbilical cord is ligated. Ampoule of 200 mg with 20 ml (10 mg/ml) starting the infusion at a rate of 2mg/kg of body weight in the first hour followed by a continuous infusion of 1mg/kg per hour until the umbilical cord ligation. Transmission of the infection from mother to child can take place at three different times:

During pregnancy: Mainly in the last weeks of gestation, during the third trimester, known as prenatal transmission. In case of acute retrovirosis during gestation, the risk of mother-to-child transmission increases by 30%.

1- During labor, or peri-natal labor: The newborn may become infested during delivery by direct exposure to the mother's blood or her fluids. Contractions of the uterus may facilitate the passage of blood from the mother to the infant.

2- Through breastfeeding, postnatal or postpartum: The risk of acquiring infection increases by 12-26% in children who are breastfed. The longer the newborn is breastfed, the higher the risk, and it is considerable after three months of age. HIV penetrates through the skin or mucous membranes of the newborn or the gastrointestinal mucosa.

The virus can be transmitted during pregnancy (mainly in late stages), there are risk factors involved in mother-to-child transmission such as):

1- Maternal factors: acute retrovirosis during gestation, duration of antiretroviral treatment, presence of STIs, nutritional status, vitamin A deficiency and maternal age.

2- Obstetric Factors

3- Viral and immunological factors

4- Factors inherent to the newborn (prematurity and low birth weight) 5- Factors related to breastfeeding (the presence of virus in breast milk is generally related to the level of viral load).

6- Psychosocial factors: smoking, intravenous drug use and unprotected sexual practices.

The nursing technician must know the criteria for the selection of the ARV regimen to be used in the HIV-positive pregnant woman.

1- Gestational age.

2- Degree of maternal

immunodeficiency. 3- Magnitude of viral

load.

4- Potential for adherence to clinical monitoring and medication use.

5- In women with CD4 greater than 250, consider the association of ARV with hepatic toxicity.

6- Take into account considerations regarding the selection of Nelfinavir or Nevirapine in the scheme.

CLARIFICATIONS ON MEDICATIONS

Nelfinavir is indicated in gestational ages below 28 weeks and in women with more marked immunosuppression.

Nevirapine offers an increased risk of severe hepatotoxicity in the first 6 weeks of treatment and requires mandatory and rigorous liver function monitoring every 15 days in the first 18 weeks and monthly follow-up after this period.

Recommendations for the use of Zidovudine in newborns

1-   Start administration of AZT oral solution in the first two hours after birth (2 mg/kg b.w. every six hours) until the sixth week (42 days).

2-   In case the newborn is not able to receive the drug orally, it should receive it by the EV route in the same dosage as the scheme recommended in point 1.

-    In the case of premature or low birth weight newborns, start with 1.5 mg/kg.

-    Prohibit breastfeeding.

Objectives

<u>**General Objective**</u>

Design a course to prepare nurses working in Primary Health Care for the management of pregnant patients living with HIV/AIDS.

<u>**Specific objectives:**</u>

1. To analyze the historical background of care for pregnant women with HIV/AIDS in Cuba and the world.
2. To determine the level of knowledge of nurses working in Primary Health Care for the management of pregnant patients living with HIV/AIDS.
3. To identify the main problems encountered by nursing personnel in the management of pregnant patients living with HIV/AIDS.

Semantic control

Gestation: It is the physiological process that begins at the moment of fertilization or conception (union of the egg with the sperm) during which a new being is formed inside the woman's uterus and ends with childbirth.

Virus: Organism unable to reproduce on its own, it depends on another cell to develop and survive.

Immunodeficiency: Impairment of the proper functioning of the body's immune system.

HIV: Human immunodeficiency virus.

AIDS: acquired immunodeficiency syndrome.

Syndrome: A group of symptoms and signs that constitute a disease.

STI: Sexually Transmitted Infection.

Antiretrovirals. Drug agents that destroy or prevent the development or multiplication of viruses. purine nucleotide analogues that inhibit replication of various RNA and DNA viruses.

Chapter 2
Theoretical Methodological Design

Methodology

A descriptive, prospective study was conducted from December 2010 to February 2011. The sample consisted of 47 nurses and nursing graduates from the Raúl Gómez Hospital polyclinic, which represents 30 percent of the nursing staff population working at the polyclinic.

<u>Inclusion parameters:</u>
Technical nurses and nursing graduates who work in the Raúl Gómez Hospital polyclinic in the care of pregnant women with HIV.

<u>Exclusion parameters:</u>

Technical nurses and nursing graduates who work in the on-call, outpatient, and departments that are not linked to the care work of the polyclinic - Raul Gomez Hospital in the care of pregnant women with HIV.

Theoretical and empirical inquiries:

The research is based on the dialectical-materialist approach that made it possible to effectively use the methods and techniques that allowed analyzing the object of study from a scientific position, to evaluate and analyze the phenomena studied in their objective, systemic character, and to reveal the internal contradictions of the object of study.

Theoretical and empirical inquiries were carried out with a dialectical materialist approach for the Theoretical Inquiries were used:

Documentary analysis: it allowed to conform the conceptual theoretical

32

framework of the research allowing the author to study the object of study and the theoretical assumptions that have been used and handled previously for the preparation of nursing personnel, the systems of improvement to which their training has been subject after graduation, and the concepts of improvement that are currently used in particular in the nursing care of pregnant patients with HIV and the consequences that affect their health and future.

Historical - logical: it made it possible to study the development process of nurses' training, studying the laws to which it has been subject and the irregularities it has presented in its historical development worldwide and in Cuba, the improvement of nurses in order to solve the professional problems related to the care of pregnant patients with HIV, the care and the professional problems faced by nurses in their professional practice to provide such care.

Comparative studies: it was used in conjunction with the historical-logical method. To study from a dialectical point of view the object of study, characterize it, the previous and current trends in the nursing care process for pregnant patients with HIV at the level of the patient.
and in Cuba, and it is possible to determine the changes that have taken place up to the present time.

Systemic approach: it allowed designing the course establishing the dialectic relationship between the theoretical basis that the nurse must have to develop the skills for the care of pregnant patients with HIV, in function of the transformation of the object of study, it allowed organizing each one of the steps through which the nurse must go through, maintaining an organicity in the development of a scientific thought,

Modeling: it was used in order to design the course that favors the optimal performance of nursing actions and the achievement of the nurses' learning for the care of pregnant patients with HIV and the satisfaction of the human needs of the population they serve during their professional practice.

Throughout the development of the research, different theoretical procedures were taken into account, such as:

Observation: it favored determining how the nursing staff performs in the process of developing professional skills for the care of pregnant patients with HIV.

Analysis and synthesis: favored the establishment of the characteristics and relationships established in the development of professional skills.

Among the empirical inquiries, the following were used:

Interview and survey, to assess whether or not a course was necessary to allow nurses to develop professional skills in an objective manner, to formulate the problem to be investigated and to develop the course, as well as to obtain knowledge about the object under investigation (pregnant patients with HIV).

Knowledge test: it was used to determine the professional problems presented by technical nurses in terms of their performance in the care of pregnant patients with HIV.

The type of research we propose to carry out is Action Research: since a self-reflective search was conducted, social research, educational work and action are integrally combined:

Research: relevance of a transformation in the professional development of nurses and their performance.

Educational work: it transforms nurses in terms of the development of professional skills, increasing their competence and performance and forming values.

Action: the implementation of the habilitation from the analysis with the medical and paramedical collective allows its transformation from its implementation.

With the use of the above inquiries, the following contributions were made:

Scientific novelty: it allows the design of a course that contributes to raising the level of preparation of nurses, the development of skills and the optimization of nursing care for pregnant patients with HIV.

Actuality: The course is a tribute to the new transformations that are taking place in our health system. The training and development of Cuban nurses not only responds at this time to the training of a professional for Cuba, but also to provide nursing care anywhere in the world, for which we must be prepared with a high scientific-technical level. The care of pregnant patients with HIV is a priority for the health system in order to improve the quality of pregnancy.

Relevance: Cuban society requires a nursing professional better prepared to successfully develop their work, in correspondence with the demands of society. The course is an alternative to overcome nurses working in primary health care (doctor's office and family nurse), in the care of pregnant patients with HIV, thus raising the level of competence and performance of nurses.

Ethical Considerations:

During the development of the research, the analysis of the results of the surveys and interviews, the general ethical considerations applicable to all research were taken into account, the anonymity and reliability of the information was maintained, respect for the right to autonomy of each nurse included in the study was maintained with informed consent.

Operationalization of variables

Variables	Ranking	Scale	Description operational
Performance	Qualitative Nominal	Assistance	Qualityof performance HIV carriers.
Competition	Qualitative Nominal	Assistance	Competencies HIV carriers

Chapter 3
Analysis and Research Results.

<u>Analysis and discussion of the results of the questionnaire application.</u>

Characterization of the nursing staff of the Raúl Gómez García polyclinic-hospital.

The polyclinic has 25 offices of the family doctor and nurse. A questionnaire was applied to identify the learning needs of the nursing staff in the management of pregnant women with HIV/AIDS and their prenatal care in the family doctor's and nurse's offices. A sample of 47 nurses was used, representing 100% of the nursing staff working at the time the questionnaire was applied. Table 1 shows the age groups in which the nursing staff at the Raúl Gómez García polyclinic-hospital is distributed, with a predominance of the 36 to 40 age group.

Table No. 1 Distribution of Nursing Personnel according to age group.

	AGE	QUANTITY	%
	20-25	1	
	26-30	5	
AGE GROUPS	31-35		
	36-40		
	41-45		
	46-50		
	TOTAL		

Source: questionnaire

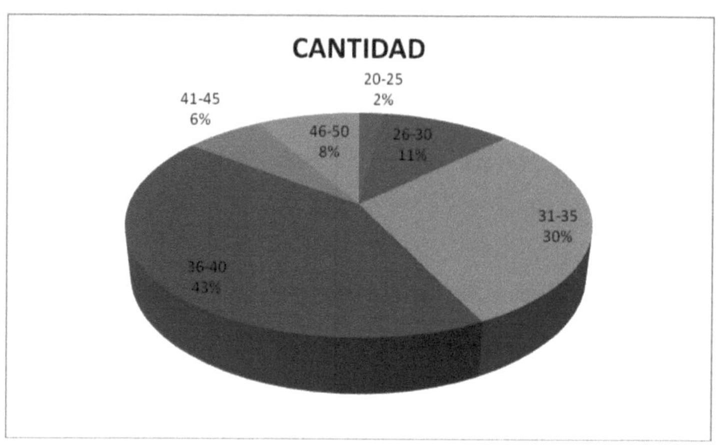

Table 2 shows the categories of nurses according to the years of graduation, showing that there is a predominance between 10-15 years with 19% and 21-25 years for 18% at the Raúl Gómez García polyclinic-hospital.

Table: 2 Characterization of the category of nurses at the Raúl Gómez García polyclinic according to years of graduation.

	QUANTITY		%
	Less than 10	1	
YEARS OF GRADUATES	10-15		
	16-20		
	21-25		
	26-30		5
	TOTAL		

Source: questionnaire

Table 3 shows the categories from the occupational point of view, with a predominance of technical nursing personnel (53.1%).

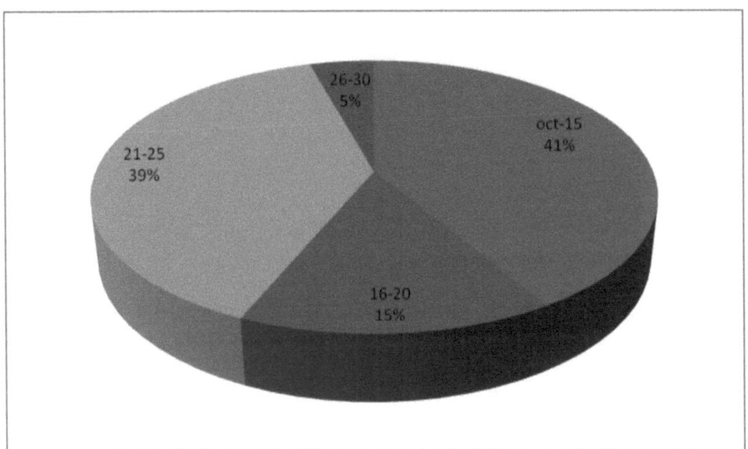

Table: 3 Characterization of the category of nurses at the Raúl Gómez García polyclinic according to their occupational category.

CATEGORY	No.	%
Bachelor of Science in Nursing		46.8
Nursing Technical Staff		53.1
TOTAL		

Source: questionnaire

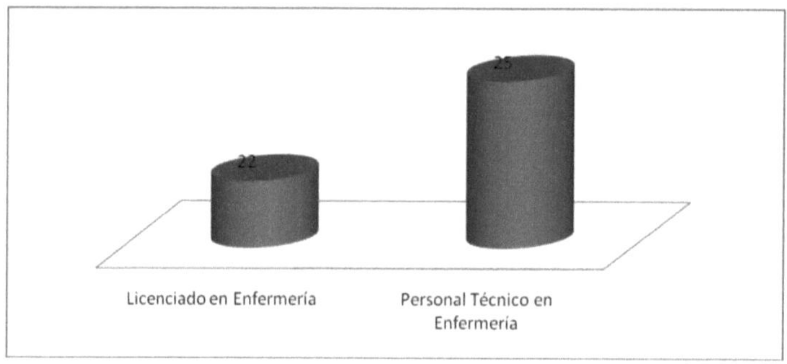

Table 4 shows the years of experience of the personnel working at the Raúl Gómez García polyclinic-hospital, showing that 40.4 percent of the personnel have worked at the Raúl Gómez García polyclinic.

The percentage corresponds to those with 10 to 15 years of experience and 38.2% are between 21 - 25 years of experience. The years of experience are important in the development of skills and intellectual capacities in the professional performance at the Raúl Gómez García polyclinic-hospital, but this does not mean that they have experience in the management of pregnant patients with HIV.

Table No. 4 Distribution of Nursing Personnel according to years of experience.

	QUANTITY		
	Years	Number	%
YEARS OF GRADUATE S	Less than 10	1	2.2
	10-15		40.4
	16-20		12.7
	21-25		38.2
	26-30		6.3
	TOTAL		

Source: questionnaire

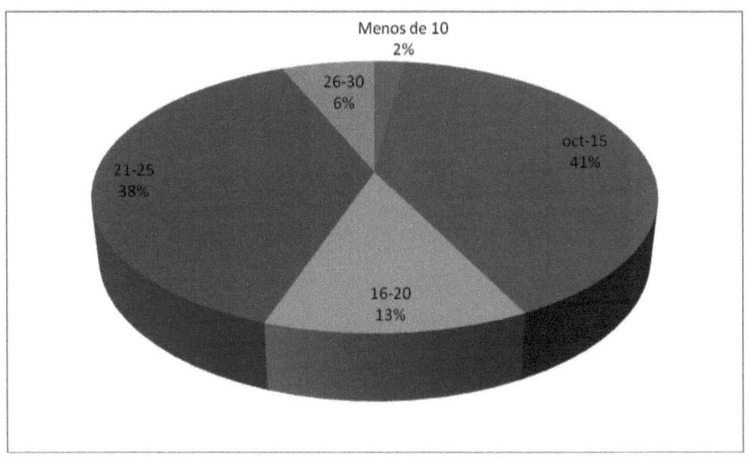

Determination of learning needs and skills in the face of pregnant patients with HIV

A knowledge test was carried out, which yielded the following results: the test showed incapacity in execution and decision making, since the correct answers about the performance of nursing personnel in the care of pregnant women with HIV were not marked: in question 1, of the 47 nurses who took the questionnaire, only 30 had knowledge about HIV, which represents 63.8%; 5 nurses knew some things, for 10.6%; and 12 nurses did not know anything, for 25.5%.

Table 5: Do you know what HIV/AIDS is?

Aspects	Yes	%	No	%	Only partially	%
1- Do you know what HIV/AIDS is?		63.8%		25.5%	5	10.6%

Source: Knowledge test

In relation to Question 2, only 46 nurses are indistinctly aware of the actions to be performed with the at-risk population, which represents 97.8%.

Table 6: Actions to be carried out with the at-risk population in health promotion and prevention activities

Aspects	Yes	%	No	%
2- Actions to be carried out with the population at risk in health promotion and prevention activities.				
a) Systematic screening of the population once a year. with risky sexual behavior.		23.4		76.6
b) Offer condoms to the population.		46.8		53.2
c) Inter-consultations with the survey nurse	-	-	-	-
d) Discuss it with family members.	-	-	1	2.1
e) Dispensing to the population with sexual conduct risk.	-	-	-	-
f) Ask for support in the CDR and FMC to control these people.		8.6		91.4
g) Educational and promotional actions, with emphasis on the use of condoms among the population of risk and evaluation of the results.	5	10.6	42	89.3
h) Work with women who are in the most vulnerable groups. risk groups and are of childbearing age.		8.5		91.4

Source: Knowledge test

In Question 3, only 39 were aware of HIV/AIDS screening groups, representing 76.6% of the nurses surveyed.

Table 7: HIV Screening Group Classification

Aspects	Yes	%	No	%
3- Classification of the HIV screening group				
a) The husband of a pregnant woman is classified in the group.				
b) Person infested with blennorrhagia lo classified in the STI group.		82.9		17.1
c) MSM requesting to undergo the study of HIV I classify it as captured.				
d) A person who voluntarily asks for the study is from the donor group.				

Source: Knowledge test

With regard to Question 4, only 36 nurses are aware of the rights of pregnant women with HIV/AIDS, which represents 76.5%.

Table 8: Rights of women of   childbearing age infected with the HIV/AIDS virus

Aspects	Yes	%	No	%
4- Rights of women of childbearing age infected with the HIV/AIDS virus				
a) Hide it				
b) Maternity		51.6		48.9
c) They have the right not to hide it		25.5		74.4
d) They are not entitled to maternity leave				
e) Do not				

Source: Knowledge test

In the analysis carried out in Question 5, only 32 nurses know that pregnant women should receive the same health services as other sick people, which represents 68.1%.

Table 9: Health services to be received by pregnant women with HIV/AIDS

Aspects	Yes	%	No	%
5- Health services that pregnant women with HIV/AIDS should receive				
More				29.7
Less			1	2.1
The Same		68.1		

Source: Knowledge test

When referring to Question 6, it is evident that only 13 nurses for a

27.6 know the management of the pregnant woman with HIV/AIDS in primary

health care

Table 10. Management of pregnant women with HIV/AIDS by the nurse in primary health care

Aspects	Yes	%	No	%	Only partially	%
6- Management of the pregnant woman with HIV/AIDS by the nurse in the care of the pregnant woman. primary health care		27.6 %		4.2 %		68.1

Source: Knowledge test

When analyzing the use of antiretroviral therapy in these patients in Question 7, out of the 47 nurses surveyed only 29 of them know the age gestational period in which the pregnant woman will receive antiretroviral treatment, which represents 61.7%.

Table 11. Gestational age for antiretroviral therapy intervention.

Aspects	Yes	%	No	%
7- Gestational age for the intervention with the antiretroviral therapy		61.7 %		38.2 %

Source: Knowledge test

In the questionnaire applied to Question 8, only 45 nurses were aware of the conduct to be followed in the care of pregnant women with HIV/AIDS, which represents 95.7%.

Table 12. Conduct to be followed in the recruitment of the HIV-positive pregnant woman.

Aspects	Yes	%	No	%
8- Conduct to be followed in the recruitment of the seropositive pregnant woman				
A) Behavior A: Alerting the partner		48.9		
B) Conduct C: Voluntary Interruption of Pregnancy		46.8		53.1

Source: Knowledge test

As shown in Question 9, only 41 nurses responded indistinctly with the antiretrovirals used in pregnancy, which represents 87.2%.

Table 13. Antiretroviral drugs used in pregnant women with HIV/AIDS

Aspects	Yes	%	No	%
9- Antiretrovirals used in pregnant women with HIV/AIDS				
a) Zidovudine		59.5		40.4
b) Nelfinavir		6.3		93.6
c) Lamivudine		21.2		78.7

Source: Knowledge test

When analyzing Table 14 in relation to question 10 of the questionnaire, it can be seen that there is a high percentage of positive responses for 63.8 of the respondents, which speaks in favor of the knowledge they have about the care they receive in other health institutions.

Table 14. Nurses' knowledge of the secondary level health institutions where specialized care is provided to HIV-positive pregnant women.

Aspects	Yes	%	No	%
10- Secondary health institutions where specialized care is provided to pregnant women with HIV/AIDS.		63.8		36.17

Source: Knowledge test

Analysis and research results

The course has great value in the improvement of nursing personnel, especially in the case of the insufficiencies detected in the needs identification process, since the contents to be worked on should be reaffirmed in these professionals and are indispensable in the current conditions in which they work, taking into account their inexperience in the management of pregnant women with HIV/AIDS. The design is based on the theory of advanced education curricular design, the theory of improvement systems and problem identification, which allowed us to fulfill the curricular dimensions.

Social dimension:

Nursing personnel working in primary health care need to be prepared to solve the health problems presented by the population, especially with regard to the care of pregnant women with HIV/AIDS. The application of principles, models and measures proposed by these theories allowed for a process of identification of needs and problems, which argues the social relevance of the project.

Psycho-educational dimension:

From the psycho-educational point of view, the project assumes a conception of learning with a historical-cultural approach in which activity and communication play a fundamental role in the training process and with which it shares the use of active methods, the use of group techniques and the attention to individual learning pace, learning needs, etc. should not only be based on the cognitive aspect but also on the study of the personality of the nurses who will receive the qualification, starting from the motivation for learning.

Philosophical dimension:

The project is based on the theory of Dialectical Materialism, both as science and method, which allowed us to determine the social needs and to know the social relevance that will support the course, in which the categories, laws and principles of dialectics are evident: unity and struggle of opposites, the transformation of qualitative changes to quantitative and vice versa, the law of negation of negation.

Epistemological Dimension:

The course was supported by the study of knowledge from the needs of appropriation of knowledge that the nursing staff had for them, which allowed the elaboration of the project in correspondence to their needs of improvement within the research work. The epistemological and historical-logical study of the course is carried out as a way of improvement, evidencing the nature of this knowledge.

Research Dimension:

Research is the fundamental link in every professional process and an elementary premise in the theory of advanced education, where it plays a determining role in encouraging the professional to search for the unknown, being present in the activities to be developed in order to achieve a high level of professionalism. In the course that we propose, research becomes the guiding thread of the whole process of complementation of this nursing staff, starting from the learning needs that the professional has to develop in order to achieve a high level of professionalism.

The medical collaborations in which the health problems differ from the Cuban context.

Advanced Education Dimension:

Advanced education as an educational paradigm is present in the whole process of the habilitated since it allows to know the human resources we have, their motivations, interests, aspirations, which will allow to enrich the proposed project, as for the proposal is based on the theory of curriculum design of advanced education.

For the elaboration of this design, the phases proposed in the theory of Advanced Education were taken into account:

- Curricular approach or design.
It was carried out based on documentary analysis and comparative studies of previous theses that dealt with the subject of pregnant women with HIV/AIDS, but in the Cuban context, which allowed the author to form the theoretical framework and reorganize the contents through modeling.

The source of information for the determination of problems was determined, and as an essential element, the level of entry of the nursing personnel was taken into account, and the system of knowledge and skills was formed from here.

The object of study was defined, which corresponds to the process of systematic organization of the course, and the general and specific objectives were elaborated for this case.

The knowledge and skills system is aimed at possessing clinical and practical skills related to the professional performance and care of pregnant women with HIV/AIDS.

The logical structure of the knowledge and skills system of the course was structured by themes that appear below.

The means and methods used in it, have implicit the methods of science in general and of the profession in particular, in the nursing care process, promoting active participation, the exchange of experience, the development of cognitive independence, the production of knowledge and consequently, creativity and skills.

The evaluation system will correspond to the objectives, through the verification of theoretical and practical knowledge, as they allow to assess their impact on professional performance, will take into account the certification and accreditation, which will be legally recognized.

Coordinator: Lic. Janet Martínez Sandrino
Professors: Principal Professors designated according to each subject.

Based on the use of modeling within the theoretical methods, it was structured taking into account the particularities of the proposed advanced evaluation form, aimed at technical nursing personnel working in emergency centers in primary health care who receive technical and practical information to treat a traumatic emergency.

Title: Propuesta de curso de capacitación sobre la atención a gestantes portadores de VIH para enfermeros que laboran en consultorios del policlínico-hospital Raúl Gómez García.

The proposed course is structured as follows:

This organizational form, typical of professional improvement and in correspondence with the Postgraduate Regulations of our country, are postgraduate figures that are not excluded and allow access to all university graduates, in order to prepare them as multipliers of this knowledge for the care of patients suffering from this disease.

General Objective:

To evaluate the management of HIV-positive pregnant women through the use of new knowledge to provide solutions to their health problems.

Entry requirements:
- ➢ Nurse Technician or Graduate Nurse
- ➢ Letter of release from the work center
- ➢ Be physically and mentally fit.
- ➢ Work in the offices of the family physician, Raúl Gómez García Polyclinic, 10 de Octubre Municipality.

COURSE STRUCTURE:

N o	TOPICS	Total Hour s	Theor etical	Practice s
1.	General information from HIV/AIDS infection			
2.	Conduct to be followed in the recruitment of the HIV-positive pregnant woman			
3.	Management of the pregnant woman with HIV/AIDS in primary health care. by the nursing staff			
4.	Intervention with antiretroviral therapy according to gestational age. Antiretrovirals most commonly used in pregnant women with HIV/AIDS.			
	TOTAL			

Teaching strategy:

This course grants a total of 3 academic credits and will be developed through the blended learning modality. The trainees will have 8 hours per week, with two frequencies per week. These will take place from 1:00 pm to 5:00 pm, in the classrooms of the Raúl Gómez García Hospital.

Lectures, workshops and seminars are among the most common forms of teaching organization. This course has as its

modality of independent work through bibliographic reviews in the hours of practical areas.

For the development of practical activities, there will be coordination with the Eusebio Hernandez Hospital and the Pedro Kouri Institute where these pregnant women with HIV are attended.

EVALUATION TOPICS:

The evaluation system includes formative and summative evaluations of all teaching and practical activities. According to the regulations of the Ministry of Higher Education, it is essential that the student has attended at least 80% of the activities.

The final evaluation of the course will consist of an integrative seminar related to one of the topics covered in the course. The evaluation will be issued as pass or fail. Upon completion and passing the course, a certificate with the corresponding total credits will be awarded.

Fundamental teaching methods

The contents of this course have a linear sequence and are used both in the theoretical and practical classes, as well as in the integrative seminar and the workshop. The classes must be previously prepared by guides, it is convenient that the professors try to develop in the practical activities the problem solving method and other active teaching methods. In the integrative seminar should be used the oriented search, the solution of problematic situations that can be known, in the method of agreeing and disagreeing the discussion of papers among others that should prevail at all times in the systemic and integrative approach of knowledge.

The seminar should try to integrate the contents of the topics with novel aspects that incorporate research results or new data of interest, preferably those related to the problems of the health area. It is the appropriate framework for the expansion and consolidation of knowledge and can be exercised in many ways.

The workshop activity is a method that is characterized predominantly by active or participatory techniques of students individually or in groups, but should be flexible and adaptable to the needs of the participants in relation to what they normally develop or will develop, where the final work is presented and evaluated, preferably as a scientific exchange in the development of the activity. The work should be oriented from the beginning, with the corresponding guidance of its design.

The teacher will act as an advisor, who will assume the framework that encompasses the process to be applied in professional nursing for the management of pregnant women with HIV/AIDS in the health area. In the workshop, the analysis of the different groups will allow consolidating and expanding knowledge and developing skills in the problem at hand Teaching Methods

In the classes, the most appropriate teaching methods consist of expository, demonstrative, questioning, discernment and group techniques that allow us to enrich the level of knowledge and skills of the student and with the use of computerization.

The seminar can use posters, computerized images and other media prepared by the nurses themselves. Especially when it is a lecture, videos related to the topic. The teaching aids in the workshop will be made, according to the determination of the strategy of the activity and the criterion of the educators in the form of a poster.

Other teaching aids:

> ➢ Electronic presentations in Power Point
> ➢ Digitized material
> ➢ Printed material
> ➢ Transparencies

Graduate Paper

The trainees will be in optimal conditions for the level of know-how in the first level of care (CMF) where the nursing professional works, allowing them to interact with the health team in the care of pregnant women with HIV/AIDS, improving the management and care of the pregnant woman, as well as in the reduction of morbidity and mortality indicators.

The acquisition of a solid and deep scientific base that allows the graduate to continuously improve the health status of the pregnant woman, by appropriating new knowledge will create the commitment of the professional with the health of the pregnant woman.

advance scientific knowledge, in favor of the development of nursing during the period that he/she works as a professional at the first level of care. Apply the scientific method of the profession, the Nursing Care Process, how to adequately manage the pregnant woman with HIV/AIDS.

Teaching Activity -1 Overview of HIV/AIDS Infection

Objectives.

1- Explain the historical background of the infection.

2- To argue the role of the nurse taking into account the anatomical-physiological alterations inherent to the infection process of the disease, in the satisfaction of the needs that may interfere with the quality of life of pregnant women.

Subject:

1.1 Concept.

1.2 Etiology.

1.3 Epidemiological chain and mechanisms of action.

1.4 Routes of transmission. Nursing actions

1.5 Natural history of infection. Classification, clinical and laboratory categories.

1.6 Role of the nurse taking into account the anatomical and physiological alterations inherent to the infection process of the disease.

Methodological Orientations

The professor will use 32 hours to develop the theoretical contents and 8 hours for the practical ones, including two hours for the round table where they will develop the role of the nurse, taking into account the anatomical-physiological alterations typical of the infection process of the disease, in the satisfaction of the needs that may interfere in the quality of life of pregnant women.

Evaluation System:

> ➢ Frequent formative evaluations:
> ➢ Conferences.
> ➢ Round tables.
> ➢ Final work.
> ➢ Preparation, delivery and discussion of a report.
> ➢ Final evaluation.
> ➢ The results achieved in the formative evaluations and the final work will be taken into account.

Teaching Activity- 2 Conduct to be followed in the recruitment of the HIV-positive pregnant woman

Objectives:

1. Apply the nursing care and follow-up algorithm for pregnant women in primary health care. 2.

Topics:

2.1   -Application of the algorithm for the follow-up of pregnant women in primary health care.

2.2   Compliance with the principles of medical ethics in the care of pregnant women.

2.3   Nursing care in the pregnancy recruitment

2.4   Epidemiological follow-up of infection in pregnant women.

Methodological Orientations

The professor will use lectures for the introduction of the new contents, will carry out a team work with the topic Compliance with the principles of medical ethics in the care of the pregnant woman, for which he will spend two hours, and at the end of the unit he will carry out an integrating seminar with an evaluative character. Of the total number of practical hours, two of them will be used for the application of Nursing Care in the pregnancy reception. The professor will evaluate the nursing care of the trainees in the presence of the patients.

Evaluation system:

❖   The final grade will be constituted by the average of the results obtained in the workshop class, the team work and the integrative seminar, in addition to the grades obtained in the frequent formative evaluations.

Teaching activity 3: Management of pregnant women with HIV/AIDS in primary health care by nurses

Objectives:

1.	Explain the role of the nurse in the integration process with secondary health care.

Topics

3.1	Nursing actions in the process of integration with secondary care.

3.2	- The role of nurses in the management of pregnant women in primary health care.

3.3	Maternal infant transmission of HIV.

Methodological Orientation

❖ The professor will teach the theoretical contents through lectures and group work. A seminar will be given for two hours respectively. The final work will consist of a practical evaluation with the patient in the performance of a nursing procedure.

Evaluation system:

    ❖ Frequent formative evaluations:

    ➢ Seminars.

    ➢ Practical classes

    ❖ Final work.

    ➢ Practical exam that will measure the knowledge acquired in the different topics of the unit.

    ❖ Final evaluation.

    ➢ The results achieved in the formative evaluations and the final work will be taken into account.

Teaching Activity 4 Intervention with antiretroviral therapy according to gestational age. Antiretrovirals most commonly used in pregnant women with HIV/AIDS **Objective:**

1.   Explain the basic aspects in the nursing action in the evaluation and management of the intoxicated person.

Topics.

4.1   - Antiretroviral drugs most commonly used in pregnancy. Form of presentation, dosage, mechanism of action, adverse reactions and precautions.

4.2   -Application of antiretroviral therapy

Methodological Orientations

The professor will use 20 hours to develop the theoretical contents and 4 hours for the practical ones, including two hours for the round table where they will develop the topic antiretroviral treatment and four hours for the final exam. Students will hand in their written work and will present it to the professor individually.

Evaluation system:

> ➢ Frequent formative evaluations:
> ➢ Conferences.
> ➢ Round tables.
> ➢ Final work.
> ➢ Preparation, delivery and discussion of a report.
> ➢ Final evaluation.

Conclusions

- The review and analysis of documents made it possible to systematize the regularities regarding postgraduate education in Cuba, the historical background of the discovery of the human immunodeficiency virus, treatment, follow-up with retrovirals and the management of pregnant women with HIV/AIDS.

- The systematization of the characterization of nurses working in primary health care made it possible to construct the dimensions, variables and indicators that made it possible to elaborate and process the instruments for the evaluation of the level of knowledge of these nurses in the management of pregnant women with HIV/AIDS.

- The analysis of the results of the empirical and theoretical inquiries made it possible to identify the problems that nurses have in caring for pregnant women with HIV/AIDS. Only 30 nurses have knowledge about HIV, which represents 63.8%, 5 nurses know some things, for 10.6%, and 12 nurses do not know, for 25.5%.

- The consideration of the theoretical and methodological foundations related to the training of Human Resources in nursing, Scientific Management and Advanced Education, is evident in the course for nurses working in primary health care (CMF), only 45 nurses know indistinctly the conduct to follow in the care of pregnant women with HIV/AIDS, which represents 95.7%.This represents 95.7% and the need for a course to improve the performance of technical nurses working in primary health care (doctor's offices and family nurse practitioners) in the management of pregnant women with HIV/AIDS.

Recommendations

- ➤ Extend the components, stages and actions of the course for the improvement of nurses in the rest of the municipalities and the province.

- ➤ Develop and apply instruments to evaluate the impact of the course.

- ➤ To increase the number of workshops and research activities on HIV/AIDS, for the benefit of the culture of nursing personnel.

- ➤ Encourage, through methodological actions, training and scientific activity, the production of didactic materials and means on HIV/AIDS.

ENTER ALGORITHM SCHEME

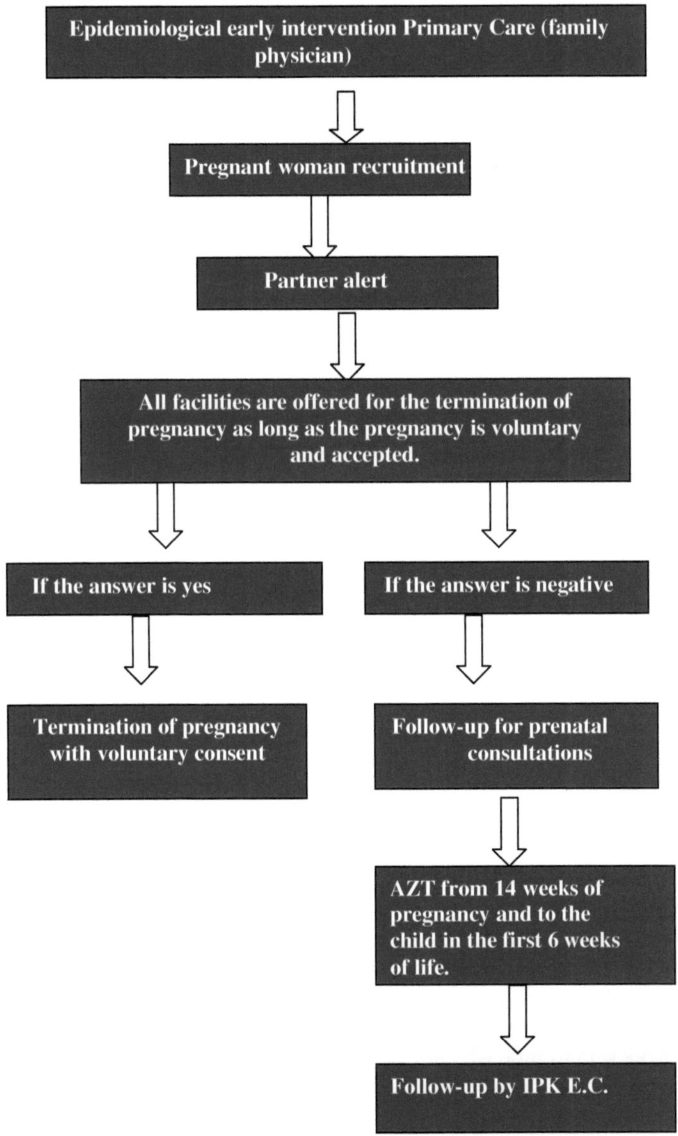

MINISTRY OF PUBLIC HEALTH

QUESTIONNAIRE
The purpose of this questionnaire is to collect information related to the learning needs that nursing personnel may have regarding the control, prevention and prenatal care of pregnant women with HIV/AIDS. It is completely anonymous and we would like it to be answered as clearly as possible.
General Data
Health Area
Occupational Category: Nurse Technician
Nurse PractitionerBachelor's Degree in Nursing
Community Nursing Specialist Maternal and Infant Nursing
Specialist
Specialist in
Intensive Nursing and
Emergency
If you are a Nurse Practitioner, please specify your age.
Sex
Graduate yearsDo you know what HIV/AIDS is?
Yes
No

Some Things
2- Taking into consideration that the work of the family physician and nurse practitioner rests on the pillars of health promotion and prevention, mark with an **X** which action(s) you would take to achieve these activities, especially with the at-risk population.
i) Systematic screening once a year of the population with risky sexual behavior.
j) Offer condoms to the population.
k) Inter-consultations with the nurse surveyor
l) Discuss with family members.
m) Dispense rizar to the population with risky sexual behavior.
n) Ask for support in the CDR and FMC to control these people.
o) Educational and promotional actions, with emphasis on the use of condoms among the population at risk and evaluation of the results.
p) Work with women who are in at-risk groups and are of childbearing age.
3- Regarding the classification of the HIV screening group. Mark the correct answer(s).
e) The husband of a pregnant woman is classified in the pregnant group.
f) A person infested with blennorrhagia is classified in the STI group.
g) MSM requesting to be tested for HIV, I classify it as captured.

h) Person who voluntarily requests the study is from the donor group.

i) MSM who frequently change partners are classified as spontaneous.

4- She thinks that women of childbearing age who know they are infected
   with the HIV/AIDS virus have the right to:

f) Hide it

g) Motherhood

h) They have the right not to hide it

i) No maternity rights

j) It is not

5- Pregnant women with HIV/AIDS. Should they receive more, less or the
   same health services as other sick people?

a)   More

Less

The same

6- Are you familiar with the management of pregnant women with HIV/AIDS
   in primary health care?

Yes

No

Some Things

7- All HIV-positive pregnant women detected in the health area will receive
    treatment with antiretroviral drugs at the first signs of infection:
    a) 5 weeks
    b) 14 weeks
    c) 10 weeks
    d) 12 weeks

8- In the recruitment of the HIV-positive pregnant woman, the conduct to be
   followed is:
    a) Partner alert
    b) Follow-up for prenatal consultations
    c) Voluntary Interruption of Pregnancy
    d) The same follow-up given to a pregnant woman who is not HIV-
        positive.

9- In HIV-positive pregnant women, the antiretroviral drugs used are:
    a) Zidovudine
    b) Nelfinavir
    c) Abacavir
    d) Lamivudine
    e) Amprenavir

10-   Do you know in which secondary health institutions specialized care
   is provided to HIV-positive pregnant women?
    Yes ____   No ____
        a) If your answer is positive, please state which ones.

INFORMED CONSENT

I hereby certify that I agree to participate in the investigation.

Once the objectives and my role in this research have been explained to me, recognizing that it does not imply risks to my personal integrity and the benefits it will bring to my professional development and to the development of this research. I have the possibility of withdrawing from the research if I consider it appropriate, without this constituting harm to my person.

For the record, I have hereunto set my hand on this day of the month of ____of the year __.

Signature _______________________________

Bibliographic references

1- Fundación Huésped, What is AIDS? [Cited: November 14, 2003] [4 screens]. Available at: http://www.huesped.org.ar/

2- Chacón Medina, Gabriela. AIDS: an analysis for adolescents. Havana, 2010

3- Phair JP, Murphy RL: Contemporary Diagnosis and Management of HIV/AIDS INFECTIONSTM. 1997. USA: 5-8

4- Orbea Espinosa, Luis Gerardo. Design of a Master's Degree Program in Comprehensive Care for People with HIV/AIDS. Aimed at Nurses, Physicians and Psychologists. National Reference Center.

5- Castro M. Evolution of Nursing in Cuba. Mimeographed Bulletin. Havana; 1999.

6- Urbina Lara, Omayda. Current Trends in Nursing Specific Competencies. National School of Public Health. Havana City. September, 2003.

7- Añorga J. The improvement of the University Teachers' Improvement System. Thesis in option to the scientific degree of Doctor in Pedagogical Sciences. Havana. MES.1989.

8- Suárez Escandón MsC. Dr. Angel. Evaluation of Toxicology Teaching in Emergency Medicine Studies. Higher Institute of Medical Sciences. Havana City, June, 2007.

Bibliography

1.   Alberto ME, Leyva HM, Vega SB, Yero A, Zamora A, Zubizarreta EM. Development alternatives for nursing personnel. In: I Iberoamerican Meeting of trainers of human resources in nursing. CENAPET. Havana; 1995.

2. Alvarez De Zayas MC. Towards a school of excellence (computer program, Windows 95: Escexc). ISPEJV. Havana; 1996.

3.   Alvarez De ZCM, Sierra V. Methodology of scientific research (computer program, Windows 95: METINV. ISPEJV. C. Havana; 1996.

4. Álvarez De ZCM. El diseño curricular en la Educación Superior Cubana (printed material). Havana; 1996.

5. Alvarez De ZRM. Towards an integral and contextualized curriculum (computer program, Windows 95: discur). ISPEJV. Havana; 1997.

6. Añorga J. The improvement of the University Teachers' Improvement System. Thesis in option to the scientific degree of Doctor in Pedagogical Sciences. Havana. MES.1989.

7.   Bello F.N, Alberto M.E, Fernández V.C, Zubizarreta E.M. Training and development of nursing human resources. A challenge for the XXI century. In: VIII SOCUENF Congress. Santiago de Cuba; 1998 May 26-29.

8. Castro M. Evolution of Nursing in Cuba. Mimeographed Bulletin. Havana; 1999.

9. Chacón Medina, Gabriela. AIDS: an analysis for adolescents. Havana, 2010

10. National Reference Workshop on Comprehensive HIV/AIDS Care. Fantasy or reality? Santiago de las Vegas. 2005.

11. Feliú, B. Et. Al. Community Nursing Model of Care.

12. Fundación Huésped, What is AIDS? [Cited: November 14, 2003] [4 screens]. Available at: http://www.huesped.org.ar/

13. Gao, SJ. Kingsley, L. Hoover, DR. Et. Al: Seroconversion to antibodies against. Kaposi's Sarcoma- Associated herpesvirus- related latent nuclear antigensbefore the development of Kaposi 's sarcoma. N, Engl. J Med-1996. Madrid. España. 1998.

14. Nursing Manual. Care of HIV seropositive persons. SSV. 15. MINSAP. Teaching and Research Area. Postgraduate studies for the

professionals in the National Health System. C. Havana; 1994.

16. MINSAP. Teaching and Research Area. Postgraduate studies for professionals in the National Health System. Havana; 1997.

17. MINSAP. Teaching and Research Area. Postgraduate Regulations in the National Health System. Havana; 1997.

18. MINSAP. CENAPEM. Study Program, Master's Degree in Medical Education. CENAPEM. Havana; 1998.

19. MINSAP. National Directorate of Nursing. Development of Scientific Degrees for university graduates in the specialty of Nursing. Methodological folder. Havana; 1998.

20. MINSAP. National Directorate of Nursing. Postgraduate Education. Methodological folder. Havana; 1997.

21. MINSAP. Plan of action for the increase of the quality of Human Resources in the National Health System. RM 142. Havana; 1996.

22. MINSAP. Regulations for the establishment of the academic credit system in the National Health System. RM 63. C. Havana; 1997. Niu, MT. Stein, DS. Schnittman, SM: Primary human immunodeficiency virus type-1 infection: Review of pathogenesis and early treatment.

intervention in human and clínical retrovirus infection. 1993. USA.

24. Orbea Espinosa, Luis Gerardo. Design of a Master's Degree Program in Comprehensive Care for People with HIV/AIDS. Aimed at Nurses, Physicians and Psychologists. National Reference Center.

25. Orbea, E, LG. Functionality of the Basic Work Group in the Center.

26. Phair JP, Murphy RL: Contemporary Diagnosis and Management of HIV/AIDS INFECTIONSTM. 1997. USA: 5-8

27. Suarez Escandon MSc. Dr. Angel. Evaluation of Toxicology Teaching in Emergency Medicine Studies. Higher Institute of Medical Sciences. Havana City, June, 2007. Nursing Union. SATSE. Occupational Health, a permanent debate.

28. Urbina Lara, Omayda. Current Trends in Nursing Specific Competencies. National School of Public Health. Havana City. September, 2003.

29. Valcárcel IN. Design of an interdisciplinary strategy of improvement for science teachers. Thesis in option to the degree of Master in Advanced Education. ISPEJV. Havana; 1996.

30. Valcárcel IN. Interdisciplinary strategy of improvement for science teachers. Thesis in option to the scientific degree of Doctor in Pedagogical Sciences. ISPEJV. Havana; 1998.

31. Vega Saumell, Berta. Postgraduate specialty program in intensivist nursing care. ISPEJV. Master's Thesis. Havana, Cuba. 1999.

32. AIDS: The epidemic of the century. A disease without a cure. [Cited: December 22, 2003]. Available at:

http://diagnostico.canal13.cl/diagnostico/html/Temas/Sida/

33. Prieto Prieto J. AIDS, chronicle and protagonists. Anti-AIDS Citizen Commission of Alava. October 30, 2003 [Cited: December 22, 2003] [8 screens]. Available at: http://www.sidalava.org/2_mod1.htm

34. Fundación Huésped, What is AIDS? [Cited: November 14, 2003] [4 screens]. Available at: http://www.huesped.org.ar/

35. Ortega González LM. Human immunodeficiency virus infection. In: Álvarez Sintes R. Temas de Medicina General Integral. Volume II. Havana: Editorial Ciencias Médicas; 2001. p. 417-21.

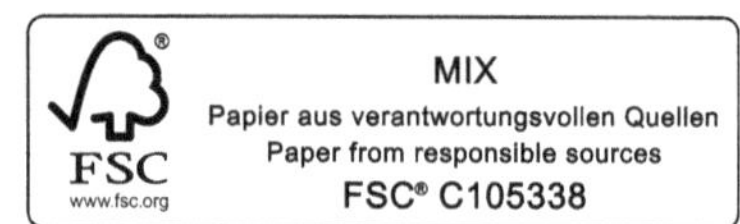

Printed by Books on Demand GmbH, Norderstedt / Germany